WORKOUT
Log Book For Men

Belongs to

Name

Adress

Phone

Start Date

End Date

Goals for Today_____ (M) (T) (W) (T) (F) (S) (S)

Muscle Group Focus _____ Weight _____ Date/Time_____

Stretch ◯ Warm-Up_____

Strength Training

Exercise	Set	1	2	3	4	5	6	7
	Reps							
	Weight							
	Reps							
	Weight							
	Reps							
	Weight							
	Reps							
	Weight							
	Reps							
	Weight							
	Reps							
	Weight							
	Reps							
	Weight							

Cardio

Exercise	Calories	Distance	Time

Water intake _____

Cooldown _____

Feeling ☆☆☆☆☆

Notes

Goals for Today_____ Ⓜ Ⓣ Ⓦ Ⓣ Ⓕ Ⓢ Ⓢ

Muscle Group Focus _____ Weight _____ Date/Time_____

Stretch ◯ Warm-Up_____

Strength Training

Exercise	Set	1	2	3	4	5	6	7
	Reps							
	Weight							
	Reps							
	Weight							
	Reps							
	Weight							
	Reps							
	Weight							
	Reps							
	Weight							
	Reps							
	Weight							
	Reps							
	Weight							
	Reps							
	Weight							

Cardio

Exercise	Calories	Distance	Time

Water intake _____

Cooldown _____

Feeling ☆☆☆☆☆

Notes

Goals for Today_____ (M) (T) (W) (T) (F) (S) (S)

Muscle Group Focus _____ Weight _____ Date/Time_____

Stretch ◯ Warm-Up_____

Strength Training

Exercise	Set	1	2	3	4	5	6	7
	Reps							
	Weight							
	Reps							
	Weight							
	Reps							
	Weight							
	Reps							
	Weight							
	Reps							
	Weight							
	Reps							
	Weight							
	Reps							
	Weight							

Cardio

Exercise	Calories	Distance	Time

Water intake _____

Cooldown _____

Feeling ☆☆☆☆☆

Notes

Goals for Today_____ Ⓜ Ⓣ Ⓦ Ⓣ Ⓕ Ⓢ Ⓢ

Muscle Group Focus _____ Weight _____ Date/Time_____

Stretch ◯ Warm-Up_____

Strength Training

Exercise	Set	1	2	3	4	5	6	7
	Reps							
	Weight							
	Reps							
	Weight							
	Reps							
	Weight							
	Reps							
	Weight							
	Reps							
	Weight							
	Reps							
	Weight							
	Reps							
	Weight							
	Reps							
	Weight							

Cardio

Exercise	Calories	Distance	Time

Water intake _____

Cooldown _____

Feeling ☆☆☆☆☆

Notes

Goals for Today_____ Ⓜ Ⓣ Ⓦ Ⓣ Ⓕ Ⓢ Ⓢ

Muscle Group Focus _____ Weight _____ Date/Time_____

Stretch ◯ Warm-Up_____

Strength Training

Exercise	Set	1	2	3	4	5	6	7
	Reps							
	Weight							
	Reps							
	Weight							
	Reps							
	Weight							
	Reps							
	Weight							
	Reps							
	Weight							
	Reps							
	Weight							
	Reps							
	Weight							
	Reps							
	Weight							

Cardio

Exercise	Calories	Distance	Time

Water intake _____

Cooldown _____

Feeling ☆☆☆☆☆

Notes

Goals for Today_____ Ⓜ Ⓣ Ⓦ Ⓣ Ⓕ Ⓢ Ⓢ

Muscle Group Focus _____ Weight _____ Date/Time_____

Stretch ◯ Warm-Up_____

Strength Training

Exercise	Set	1	2	3	4	5	6	7
	Reps							
	Weight							
	Reps							
	Weight							
	Reps							
	Weight							
	Reps							
	Weight							
	Reps							
	Weight							
	Reps							
	Weight							
	Reps							
	Weight							
	Reps							
	Weight							

Cardio

Exercise	Calories	Distance	Time
_____			____
_____			
_____			
_____			____

Water intake _____

Cooldown _____

Feeling ☆☆☆☆☆

Notes

Goals for Today_____ Ⓜ Ⓣ Ⓦ Ⓣ Ⓕ Ⓢ Ⓢ

Muscle Group Focus _____ Weight _____ Date/Time_____

Stretch ◯ Warm-Up_____

Strength Training

Exercise	Set	1	2	3	4	5	6	7
	Reps							
	Weight							
	Reps							
	Weight							
	Reps							
	Weight							
	Reps							
	Weight							
	Reps							
	Weight							
	Reps							
	Weight							
	Reps							
	Weight							

Cardio

Exercise	Calories	Distance	Time

Water intake _____

Cooldown _____

Feeling ☆☆☆☆☆

Notes

Goals for Today_____   Ⓜ Ⓣ Ⓦ Ⓣ Ⓕ Ⓢ Ⓢ

Muscle Group Focus _____ Weight _____ Date/Time_____

Stretch ◯   Warm-Up_____

Strength Training

Exercise	Set	1	2	3	4	5	6	7
	Reps							
	Weight							
	Reps							
	Weight							
	Reps							
	Weight							
	Reps							
	Weight							
	Reps							
	Weight							
	Reps							
	Weight							
	Reps							
	Weight							
	Reps							
	Weight							

Cardio

Exercise	Calories	Distance	Time
_____			
_____			
_____			
_____			

Water intake _____

Cooldown _____

Feeling ☆☆☆☆☆

Notes

[   ]

Goals for Today_____ (M) (T) (W) (T) (F) (S) (S)

Muscle Group Focus _____ Weight _____ Date/Time_____

Stretch ◯ Warm-Up_____

Strength Training

Exercise	Set	1	2	3	4	5	6	7
	Reps							
	Weight							
	Reps							
	Weight							
	Reps							
	Weight							
	Reps							
	Weight							
	Reps							
	Weight							
	Reps							
	Weight							
	Reps							
	Weight							

Cardio

Exercise	Calories	Distance	Time

Water intake _____

Cooldown _____

Feeling ☆☆☆☆☆

Notes

Goals for Today_____ Ⓜ Ⓣ Ⓦ Ⓣ Ⓕ Ⓢ Ⓢ

Muscle Group Focus _____ Weight _____ Date/Time_____

Stretch ◯ Warm-Up_____

Strength Training

Exercise	Set	1	2	3	4	5	6	7
	Reps							
	Weight							
	Reps							
	Weight							
	Reps							
	Weight							
	Reps							
	Weight							
	Reps							
	Weight							
	Reps							
	Weight							
	Reps							
	Weight							
	Reps							
	Weight							

Cardio

Exercise	Calories	Distance	Time

Water intake _____

Cooldown _____

Feeling ☆☆☆☆☆

Notes

Body Measurement

Date/Period						
Weight						
Body Fat %						
Neck						
Shoulders						
Chest						
Bicep Right						
Bicep Left						
Forearm Right						
Forearm Left						
Wrist						
Waist						
Hips						
Thigh Right						
Thigh Left						
Calf Right						
Calf Left						

Goals

Description	Deadline

Goals for Today_____ (M) (T) (W) (T) (F) (S) (S)

Muscle Group Focus _____ Weight _____ Date/Time_____

Stretch ◯ Warm-Up_____

Strength Training

Exercise	Set	1	2	3	4	5	6	7
	Reps							
	Weight							
	Reps							
	Weight							
	Reps							
	Weight							
	Reps							
	Weight							
	Reps							
	Weight							
	Reps							
	Weight							
	Reps							
	Weight							
	Reps							
	Weight							

Cardio

Exercise	Calories	Distance	Time

Water intake _____

Cooldown _____

Feeling ☆☆☆☆☆

Notes

Goals for Today_____ (M) (T) (W) (T) (F) (S) (S)

Muscle Group Focus _____ Weight _____ Date/Time_____

Stretch ◯ Warm-Up_____

Strength Training

Exercise	Set	1	2	3	4	5	6	7
	Reps							
	Weight							
	Reps							
	Weight							
	Reps							
	Weight							
	Reps							
	Weight							
	Reps							
	Weight							
	Reps							
	Weight							
	Reps							
	Weight							
	Reps							
	Weight							

Cardio

Exercise

	Calories	Distance	Time

Water intake _____

Cooldown _____

Feeling ☆☆☆☆☆

Notes

Goals for Today_____ (M) (T) (W) (T) (F) (S) (S)

Muscle Group Focus _____ Weight _____ Date/Time_____

Stretch ○ Warm-Up_____

Strength Training

Exercise	Set	1	2	3	4	5	6	7
	Reps							
	Weight							
	Reps							
	Weight							
	Reps							
	Weight							
	Reps							
	Weight							
	Reps							
	Weight							
	Reps							
	Weight							
	Reps							
	Weight							
	Reps							
	Weight							

Cardio

Exercise	Calories	Distance	Time

Water intake _____

Cooldown _____

Feeling ☆☆☆☆☆

Notes

Goals for Today_____ Ⓜ Ⓣ Ⓦ Ⓣ Ⓕ Ⓢ Ⓢ

Muscle Group Focus _____ Weight _____ Date/Time_____

Stretch ◯ Warm-Up_____

Strength Training

Exercise	Set	1	2	3	4	5	6	7
	Reps							
	Weight							
	Reps							
	Weight							
	Reps							
	Weight							
	Reps							
	Weight							
	Reps							
	Weight							
	Reps							
	Weight							
	Reps							
	Weight							
	Reps							
	Weight							

Cardio

Exercise	Calories	Distance	Time

Water intake _____

Cooldown _____

Feeling ☆☆☆☆☆

Notes

Goals for Today_____ (M) (T) (W) (T) (F) (S) (S)

Muscle Group Focus _____ Weight _____ Date/Time_____

Stretch ◯ Warm-Up_____

Strength Training

Exercise	Set	1	2	3	4	5	6	7
	Reps							
	Weight							
	Reps							
	Weight							
	Reps							
	Weight							
	Reps							
	Weight							
	Reps							
	Weight							
	Reps							
	Weight							
	Reps							
	Weight							
	Reps							
	Weight							

Cardio

Exercise	Calories	Distance	Time

Water intake _____

Cooldown _____

Feeling ☆☆☆☆☆

Notes

Goals for Today_____ (M) (T) (W) (T) (F) (S) (S)

Muscle Group Focus _____ Weight _____ Date/Time_____

Stretch ◯   Warm-Up_____

Strength Training

Exercise	Set	1	2	3	4	5	6	7
	Reps							
	Weight							
	Reps							
	Weight							
	Reps							
	Weight							
	Reps							
	Weight							
	Reps							
	Weight							
	Reps							
	Weight							
	Reps							
	Weight							
	Reps							
	Weight							

Cardio

Exercise	Calories	Distance	Time

Water intake _____

Cooldown _____

Feeling ☆☆☆☆☆

Notes

Goals for Today_____ (M) (T) (W) (T) (F) (S) (S)

Muscle Group Focus _____ Weight _____ Date/Time_____

Stretch ○ Warm-Up_____

Strength Training

Exercise	Set	1	2	3	4	5	6	7
	Reps							
	Weight							
	Reps							
	Weight							
	Reps							
	Weight							
	Reps							
	Weight							
	Reps							
	Weight							
	Reps							
	Weight							
	Reps							
	Weight							

Cardio

Exercise	Calories	Distance	Time

Water intake _____

Cooldown _____

Feeling ☆☆☆☆☆

Notes

Goals for Today_____ (M) (T) (W) (T) (F) (S) (S)

Muscle Group Focus _____ Weight _____ Date/Time_____

Stretch ◯   Warm-Up_____

Strength Training

Exercise	Set	1	2	3	4	5	6	7
	Reps							
	Weight							
	Reps							
	Weight							
	Reps							
	Weight							
	Reps							
	Weight							
	Reps							
	Weight							
	Reps							
	Weight							
	Reps							
	Weight							
	Reps							
	Weight							

Cardio

Exercise	Calories	Distance	Time

Water intake _____

Cooldown _____

Feeling ☆☆☆☆☆

Notes

Goals for Today_____ (M) (T) (W) (T) (F) (S) (S)

Muscle Group Focus _____ Weight _____ Date/Time_____

Stretch ○ Warm-Up_____

Strength Training

Exercise	Set	1	2	3	4	5	6	7
	Reps							
	Weight							
	Reps							
	Weight							
	Reps							
	Weight							
	Reps							
	Weight							
	Reps							
	Weight							
	Reps							
	Weight							
	Reps							
	Weight							

Cardio

Exercise	Calories	Distance	Time

Water intake _____

Cooldown _____

Feeling ☆☆☆☆☆

Notes

Goals for Today_____   Ⓜ Ⓣ Ⓦ Ⓣ Ⓕ Ⓢ Ⓢ

Muscle Group Focus _____ Weight _____ Date/Time_____

Stretch ◯ Warm-Up_____

Strength Training

Exercise	Set	1	2	3	4	5	6	7
	Reps							
	Weight							
	Reps							
	Weight							
	Reps							
	Weight							
	Reps							
	Weight							
	Reps							
	Weight							
	Reps							
	Weight							
	Reps							
	Weight							
	Reps							
	Weight							

Cardio

Exercise	Calories	Distance	Time
_____			_____
_____			_____
_____			_____
_____			_____

Water intake _____

Cooldown _____

Feeling ☆☆☆☆☆

Notes

Body Measurement

Date/Period						
Weight						
Body Fat %						
Neck						
Shoulders						
Chest						
Bicep Right						
Bicep Left						
Forearm Right						
Forearm Left						
Wrist						
Waist						
Hips						
Thigh Right						
Thigh Left						
Calf Right						
Calf Left						

Goals

Description	Deadline

Goals for Today_____   (M) (T) (W) (T) (F) (S) (S)

Muscle Group Focus _____ Weight _____ Date/Time_____

Stretch ◯   Warm-Up_____

Strength Training

Exercise	Set	1	2	3	4	5	6	7
	Reps							
	Weight							
	Reps							
	Weight							
	Reps							
	Weight							
	Reps							
	Weight							
	Reps							
	Weight							
	Reps							
	Weight							
	Reps							
	Weight							
	Reps							
	Weight							

Cardio

Exercise	Calories	Distance	Time

Water intake _____

Cooldown _____

Feeling ☆☆☆☆☆

Notes

Goals for Today_____ Ⓜ Ⓣ Ⓦ Ⓣ Ⓕ Ⓢ Ⓢ

Muscle Group Focus _____ Weight _____ Date/Time_____

Stretch ◯ Warm-Up_____

Strength Training

Exercise	Set	1	2	3	4	5	6	7
	Reps							
	Weight							
	Reps							
	Weight							
	Reps							
	Weight							
	Reps							
	Weight							
	Reps							
	Weight							
	Reps							
	Weight							
	Reps							
	Weight							
	Reps							
	Weight							

Cardio

Exercise	Calories	Distance	Time

Water intake _____

Cooldown _____

Feeling ☆☆☆☆☆

Notes

Goals for Today_____ (M) (T) (W) (T) (F) (S) (S)

Muscle Group Focus _____ Weight _____ Date/Time_____

Stretch ◯ Warm-Up_____

Strength Training

Exercise	Set	1	2	3	4	5	6	7
	Reps							
	Weight							
	Reps							
	Weight							
	Reps							
	Weight							
	Reps							
	Weight							
	Reps							
	Weight							
	Reps							
	Weight							
	Reps							
	Weight							
	Reps							
	Weight							

Cardio

Exercise	Calories	Distance	Time

Water intake _____

Cooldown _____

Feeling ☆☆☆☆☆

Notes

Goals for Today_____ (M) (T) (W) (T) (F) (S) (S)

Muscle Group Focus _____ Weight _____ Date/Time_____

Stretch ◯ Warm-Up_____

Strength Training

Exercise	Set	1	2	3	4	5	6	7
	Reps							
	Weight							
	Reps							
	Weight							
	Reps							
	Weight							
	Reps							
	Weight							
	Reps							
	Weight							
	Reps							
	Weight							
	Reps							
	Weight							
	Reps							
	Weight							

Cardio

Exercise	Calories	Distance	Time

Water intake _____

Cooldown _____

Feeling ☆☆☆☆☆

Notes

Goals for Today_____ (M) (T) (W) (T) (F) (S) (S)

Muscle Group Focus _____ Weight _____ Date/Time_____

Stretch ◯ Warm-Up_____

Strength Training

Exercise	Set	1	2	3	4	5	6	7
	Reps							
	Weight							
	Reps							
	Weight							
	Reps							
	Weight							
	Reps							
	Weight							
	Reps							
	Weight							
	Reps							
	Weight							
	Reps							
	Weight							
	Reps							
	Weight							

Cardio

Exercise	Calories	Distance	Time

Water intake _____

Cooldown _____

Feeling ☆☆☆☆☆

Notes

Goals for Today_____ Ⓜ Ⓣ Ⓦ Ⓣ Ⓕ Ⓢ Ⓢ

Muscle Group Focus _____ Weight _____ Date/Time_____

Stretch ◯ Warm-Up_____

Strength Training

Exercise	Set	1	2	3	4	5	6	7
	Reps							
	Weight							
	Reps							
	Weight							
	Reps							
	Weight							
	Reps							
	Weight							
	Reps							
	Weight							
	Reps							
	Weight							
	Reps							
	Weight							
	Reps							
	Weight							

Cardio

Exercise	Calories	Distance	Time

Water intake _____

Cooldown _____

Feeling ☆☆☆☆☆

Notes

Goals for Today_____ Ⓜ Ⓣ Ⓦ Ⓣ Ⓕ Ⓢ Ⓢ

Muscle Group Focus _____ Weight _____ Date/Time_____

Stretch ○ Warm-Up_____

Strength Training

Exercise	Set	1	2	3	4	5	6	7
	Reps							
	Weight							
	Reps							
	Weight							
	Reps							
	Weight							
	Reps							
	Weight							
	Reps							
	Weight							
	Reps							
	Weight							
	Reps							
	Weight							
	Reps							
	Weight							

Cardio

Exercise	Calories	Distance	Time

Water intake _____

Cooldown _____

Feeling ☆☆☆☆☆

Notes

Goals for Today_____ Ⓜ Ⓣ Ⓦ Ⓣ Ⓕ Ⓢ Ⓢ

Muscle Group Focus _____ Weight _____ Date/Time_____

Stretch ◯ Warm-Up_____

Strength Training

Exercise	Set	1	2	3	4	5	6	7
	Reps							
	Weight							
	Reps							
	Weight							
	Reps							
	Weight							
	Reps							
	Weight							
	Reps							
	Weight							
	Reps							
	Weight							
	Reps							
	Weight							
	Reps							
	Weight							

Cardio

Exercise	Calories	Distance	Time

Water intake _____

Cooldown _____

Feeling ☆☆☆☆☆

Notes

Goals for Today_____ Ⓜ Ⓣ Ⓦ Ⓣ Ⓕ Ⓢ Ⓢ

Muscle Group Focus _____ Weight _____ Date/Time_____

Stretch ○ Warm-Up_____

Strength Training

Exercise	Set	1	2	3	4	5	6	7
	Reps							
	Weight							
	Reps							
	Weight							
	Reps							
	Weight							
	Reps							
	Weight							
	Reps							
	Weight							
	Reps							
	Weight							
	Reps							
	Weight							

Cardio

Exercise	Calories	Distance	Time

Water intake _____

Cooldown _____

Feeling ☆☆☆☆☆

Notes

Goals for Today_____ Ⓜ Ⓣ Ⓦ Ⓣ Ⓕ Ⓢ Ⓢ

Muscle Group Focus _____ Weight _____ Date/Time_____

Stretch ◯ Warm-Up_____

Strength Training

Exercise	Set	1	2	3	4	5	6	7
	Reps							
	Weight							
	Reps							
	Weight							
	Reps							
	Weight							
	Reps							
	Weight							
	Reps							
	Weight							
	Reps							
	Weight							
	Reps							
	Weight							
	Reps							
	Weight							

Cardio

Exercise	Calories	Distance	Time

Water intake _____

Cooldown _____

Feeling ☆☆☆☆☆

Notes

Body Measurement

Date/Period						
Weight						
Body Fat %						
Neck						
Shoulders						
Chest						
Bicep Right						
Bicep Left						
Forearm Right						
Forearm Left						
Wrist						
Waist						
Hips						
Thigh Right						
Thigh Left						
Calf Right						
Calf Left						

Goals

Description	Deadline

Goals for Today_____ Ⓜ Ⓣ Ⓦ Ⓣ Ⓕ Ⓢ Ⓢ

Muscle Group Focus _____ Weight _____ Date/Time_____

Stretch ◯ Warm-Up_____

Strength Training

Exercise	Set	1	2	3	4	5	6	7
	Reps							
	Weight							
	Reps							
	Weight							
	Reps							
	Weight							
	Reps							
	Weight							
	Reps							
	Weight							
	Reps							
	Weight							
	Reps							
	Weight							

Cardio

Exercise	Calories	Distance	Time

Water intake _____

Cooldown _____

Feeling ☆☆☆☆☆

Notes

Goals for Today_____ Ⓜ Ⓣ Ⓦ Ⓣ Ⓕ Ⓢ Ⓢ

Muscle Group Focus _____ Weight _____ Date/Time_____

Stretch ◯ Warm-Up_____

Strength Training

Exercise	Set	1	2	3	4	5	6	7
	Reps							
	Weight							
	Reps							
	Weight							
	Reps							
	Weight							
	Reps							
	Weight							
	Reps							
	Weight							
	Reps							
	Weight							
	Reps							
	Weight							
	Reps							
	Weight							

Cardio

Exercise	Calories	Distance	Time

Water intake _____

Cooldown _____

Feeling ☆☆☆☆☆

Notes

Goals for Today_____ Ⓜ Ⓣ Ⓦ Ⓣ Ⓕ Ⓢ Ⓢ

Muscle Group Focus _____ Weight _____ Date/Time_____

Stretch ◯ Warm-Up_____

Strength Training

Exercise	Set	1	2	3	4	5	6	7
	Reps							
	Weight							
	Reps							
	Weight							
	Reps							
	Weight							
	Reps							
	Weight							
	Reps							
	Weight							
	Reps							
	Weight							
	Reps							
	Weight							
	Reps							
	Weight							

Cardio

Exercise	Calories	Distance	Time

Water intake _____

Cooldown _____

Feeling ☆☆☆☆☆

Notes

Goals for Today_____ (M) (T) (W) (T) (F) (S) (S)

Muscle Group Focus _____ Weight _____ Date/Time_____

Stretch ○ Warm-Up_____

Strength Training

Exercise	Set	1	2	3	4	5	6	7
	Reps							
	Weight							
	Reps							
	Weight							
	Reps							
	Weight							
	Reps							
	Weight							
	Reps							
	Weight							
	Reps							
	Weight							
	Reps							
	Weight							
	Reps							
	Weight							

Cardio

Exercise	Calories	Distance	Time

Water intake _____

Cooldown _____

Feeling ☆☆☆☆☆

Notes

Goals for Today_____ Ⓜ Ⓣ Ⓦ Ⓣ Ⓕ Ⓢ Ⓢ

Muscle Group Focus _____ Weight _____ Date/Time_____

Stretch ◯ Warm-Up_____

Strength Training

Exercise	Set	1	2	3	4	5	6	7
	Reps							
	Weight							
	Reps							
	Weight							
	Reps							
	Weight							
	Reps							
	Weight							
	Reps							
	Weight							
	Reps							
	Weight							
	Reps							
	Weight							
	Reps							
	Weight							

Cardio

Exercise	Calories	Distance	Time

Water intake _____

Cooldown _____

Feeling ☆☆☆☆☆

Notes

Goals for Today_____ Ⓜ Ⓣ Ⓦ Ⓣ Ⓕ Ⓢ Ⓢ

Muscle Group Focus _____ Weight _____ Date/Time_____

Stretch ◯   Warm-Up_____

Strength Training

Exercise	Set	1	2	3	4	5	6	7
	Reps							
	Weight							
	Reps							
	Weight							
	Reps							
	Weight							
	Reps							
	Weight							
	Reps							
	Weight							
	Reps							
	Weight							
	Reps							
	Weight							
	Reps							
	Weight							

Cardio

Exercise	Calories	Distance	Time

Water intake _____

Cooldown _____

Feeling ☆☆☆☆☆

Notes

Goals for Today_____ (M) (T) (W) (T) (F) (S) (S)

Muscle Group Focus _____ Weight _____ Date/Time_____

Stretch ◯ Warm-Up_____

Strength Training

Exercise	Set	1	2	3	4	5	6	7
	Reps							
	Weight							
	Reps							
	Weight							
	Reps							
	Weight							
	Reps							
	Weight							
	Reps							
	Weight							
	Reps							
	Weight							
	Reps							
	Weight							

Cardio

Exercise	Calories	Distance	Time

Water intake _____

Cooldown _____

Feeling ☆☆☆☆☆

Notes

Goals for Today_____ (M) (T) (W) (T) (F) (S) (S)

Muscle Group Focus _____ Weight _____ Date/Time_____

Stretch ○ Warm-Up_____

Strength Training

Exercise	Set	1	2	3	4	5	6	7
	Reps							
	Weight							
	Reps							
	Weight							
	Reps							
	Weight							
	Reps							
	Weight							
	Reps							
	Weight							
	Reps							
	Weight							
	Reps							
	Weight							
	Reps							
	Weight							

Cardio

Exercise	Calories	Distance	Time

Water intake _____

Cooldown _____

Feeling ☆☆☆☆☆

Notes

Goals for Today_____ Ⓜ Ⓣ Ⓦ Ⓣ Ⓕ Ⓢ Ⓢ

Muscle Group Focus _____ Weight _____ Date/Time_____

Stretch ◯ Warm-Up_____

Strength Training

Exercise	Set	1	2	3	4	5	6	7
	Reps							
	Weight							
	Reps							
	Weight							
	Reps							
	Weight							
	Reps							
	Weight							
	Reps							
	Weight							
	Reps							
	Weight							
	Reps							
	Weight							
	Reps							
	Weight							

Cardio

Exercise

	Calories	Distance	Time
_____			
_____			
_____			
_____			

Water intake _____

Cooldown _____

Feeling ☆☆☆☆☆

Notes

Goals for Today_____ Ⓜ Ⓣ Ⓦ Ⓣ Ⓕ Ⓢ Ⓢ

Muscle Group Focus _____ Weight _____ Date/Time_____

Stretch ◯ Warm-Up_____

Strength Training

Exercise	Set	1	2	3	4	5	6	7
	Reps							
	Weight							
	Reps							
	Weight							
	Reps							
	Weight							
	Reps							
	Weight							
	Reps							
	Weight							
	Reps							
	Weight							
	Reps							
	Weight							
	Reps							
	Weight							

Cardio

Exercise	Calories	Distance	Time

Water intake _____

Cooldown _____

Feeling ☆☆☆☆☆

Notes

Body Measurement

Date/Period						
Weight						
Body Fat %						
Neck						
Shoulders						
Chest						
Bicep Right						
Bicep Left						
Forearm Right						
Forearm Left						
Wrist						
Waist						
Hips						
Thigh Right						
Thigh Left						
Calf Right						
Calf Left						

Goals

Description	Deadline

Goals for Today_____ (M) (T) (W) (T) (F) (S) (S)

Muscle Group Focus _____ Weight _____ Date/Time_____

Stretch ◯ Warm-Up_____

Strength Training

Exercise	Set	1	2	3	4	5	6	7
	Reps							
	Weight							
	Reps							
	Weight							
	Reps							
	Weight							
	Reps							
	Weight							
	Reps							
	Weight							
	Reps							
	Weight							
	Reps							
	Weight							
	Reps							
	Weight							

Cardio

Exercise	Calories	Distance	Time

Water intake _____

Cooldown _____

Feeling ☆☆☆☆☆

Notes

Goals for Today_____ Ⓜ Ⓣ Ⓦ Ⓣ Ⓕ Ⓢ Ⓢ

Muscle Group Focus _____ Weight _____ Date/Time_____

Stretch ◯ Warm-Up_____

Strength Training

Exercise	Set	1	2	3	4	5	6	7
	Reps							
	Weight							
	Reps							
	Weight							
	Reps							
	Weight							
	Reps							
	Weight							
	Reps							
	Weight							
	Reps							
	Weight							
	Reps							
	Weight							
	Reps							
	Weight							

Cardio

Exercise	Calories	Distance	Time

Water intake _____

Cooldown _____

Feeling ☆☆☆☆☆

Notes

Goals for Today_____ Ⓜ Ⓣ Ⓦ Ⓣ Ⓕ Ⓢ Ⓢ

Muscle Group Focus _____ Weight _____ Date/Time_____

Stretch ◯ Warm-Up_____

Strength Training

Exercise	Set	1	2	3	4	5	6	7
	Reps							
	Weight							
	Reps							
	Weight							
	Reps							
	Weight							
	Reps							
	Weight							
	Reps							
	Weight							
	Reps							
	Weight							
	Reps							
	Weight							
	Reps							
	Weight							

Cardio

Exercise	Calories	Distance	Time

Water intake _____

Cooldown _____

Feeling ☆☆☆☆☆

Notes

Goals for Today_____ Ⓜ Ⓣ Ⓦ Ⓣ Ⓕ Ⓢ Ⓢ

Muscle Group Focus _____ Weight _____ Date/Time_____

Stretch ○ Warm-Up_____

Strength Training

Exercise	Set	1	2	3	4	5	6	7
	Reps							
	Weight							
	Reps							
	Weight							
	Reps							
	Weight							
	Reps							
	Weight							
	Reps							
	Weight							
	Reps							
	Weight							
	Reps							
	Weight							
	Reps							
	Weight							

Cardio

Exercise	Calories	Distance	Time

Water intake _____

Cooldown _____

Feeling ☆☆☆☆☆

Notes

Goals for Today_____ Ⓜ Ⓣ Ⓦ Ⓣ Ⓕ Ⓢ Ⓢ

Muscle Group Focus _____ Weight _____ Date/Time_____

Stretch ◯ Warm-Up_____

Strength Training

Exercise	Set	1	2	3	4	5	6	7
	Reps							
	Weight							
	Reps							
	Weight							
	Reps							
	Weight							
	Reps							
	Weight							
	Reps							
	Weight							
	Reps							
	Weight							
	Reps							
	Weight							
	Reps							
	Weight							

Cardio

Exercise	Calories	Distance	Time

Water intake _____

Cooldown _____

Feeling ☆☆☆☆☆

Notes

Goals for Today_____ Ⓜ Ⓣ Ⓦ Ⓣ Ⓕ Ⓢ Ⓢ

Muscle Group Focus _____ Weight _____ Date/Time_____

Stretch ◯   Warm-Up_____

Strength Training

Exercise	Set	1	2	3	4	5	6	7
	Reps							
	Weight							
	Reps							
	Weight							
	Reps							
	Weight							
	Reps							
	Weight							
	Reps							
	Weight							
	Reps							
	Weight							
	Reps							
	Weight							
	Reps							
	Weight							

Cardio

Exercise	Calories	Distance	Time

Water intake _____

Cooldown _____

Feeling ☆☆☆☆☆

Notes

Goals for Today_____ (M) (T) (W) (T) (F) (S) (S)

Muscle Group Focus _____ Weight _____ Date/Time_____

Stretch ◯ Warm-Up_____

Strength Training

Exercise	Set	1	2	3	4	5	6	7
	Reps							
	Weight							
	Reps							
	Weight							
	Reps							
	Weight							
	Reps							
	Weight							
	Reps							
	Weight							
	Reps							
	Weight							
	Reps							
	Weight							
	Reps							
	Weight							

Cardio

Exercise	Calories	Distance	Time

Water intake _____

Cooldown _____

Feeling ☆☆☆☆☆

Notes

Goals for Today_____ (M) (T) (W) (T) (F) (S) (S)

Muscle Group Focus _____ Weight _____ Date/Time_____

Stretch ◯ Warm-Up_____

Strength Training

Exercise	Set	1	2	3	4	5	6	7
	Reps							
	Weight							
	Reps							
	Weight							
	Reps							
	Weight							
	Reps							
	Weight							
	Reps							
	Weight							
	Reps							
	Weight							
	Reps							
	Weight							
	Reps							
	Weight							

Cardio

Exercise	Calories	Distance	Time

Water intake _____

Cooldown _____

Feeling ☆☆☆☆☆

Notes

Goals for Today_____   Ⓜ Ⓣ Ⓦ Ⓣ Ⓕ Ⓢ Ⓢ

Muscle Group Focus _____   Weight _____ Date/Time_____

Stretch ○ Warm-Up_____

Strength Training

Exercise	Set	1	2	3	4	5	6	7
	Reps							
	Weight							
	Reps							
	Weight							
	Reps							
	Weight							
	Reps							
	Weight							
	Reps							
	Weight							
	Reps							
	Weight							
	Reps							
	Weight							
	Reps							
	Weight							

Cardio

Exercise	Calories	Distance	Time

Water intake _____

Cooldown _____

Feeling ☆☆☆☆☆

Notes

Goals for Today_____ (M) (T) (W) (T) (F) (S) (S)

Muscle Group Focus _____ Weight _____ Date/Time_____

Stretch ◯ Warm-Up_____

Strength Training

Exercise	Set	1	2	3	4	5	6	7
	Reps							
	Weight							
	Reps							
	Weight							
	Reps							
	Weight							
	Reps							
	Weight							
	Reps							
	Weight							
	Reps							
	Weight							
	Reps							
	Weight							
	Reps							
	Weight							

Cardio

Exercise	Calories	Distance	Time

Water intake _____

Cooldown _____

Feeling ☆☆☆☆☆

Notes

Body Measurement

Date/Period						
Weight						
Body Fat %						
Neck						
Shoulders						
Chest						
Bicep Right						
Bicep Left						
Forearm Right						
Forearm Left						
Wrist						
Waist						
Hips						
Thigh Right						
Thigh Left						
Calf Right						
Calf Left						

Goals

Description	Deadline

Goals for Today_____ (M) (T) (W) (T) (F) (S) (S)

Muscle Group Focus _____ Weight _____ Date/Time_____

Stretch ◯ Warm-Up_____

Strength Training

Exercise	Set	1	2	3	4	5	6	7
	Reps							
	Weight							
	Reps							
	Weight							
	Reps							
	Weight							
	Reps							
	Weight							
	Reps							
	Weight							
	Reps							
	Weight							
	Reps							
	Weight							

Cardio

Exercise	Calories	Distance	Time

Water intake _____

Cooldown _____

Feeling ☆☆☆☆☆

Notes

Goals for Today_____ Ⓜ Ⓣ Ⓦ Ⓣ Ⓕ Ⓢ Ⓢ

Muscle Group Focus _____ Weight _____ Date/Time_____

Stretch ◯ Warm-Up_____

Strength Training

Exercise	Set	1	2	3	4	5	6	7
	Reps							
	Weight							
	Reps							
	Weight							
	Reps							
	Weight							
	Reps							
	Weight							
	Reps							
	Weight							
	Reps							
	Weight							
	Reps							
	Weight							
	Reps							
	Weight							

Cardio

Exercise	Calories	Distance	Time

Water intake _____

Cooldown _____

Feeling ☆☆☆☆☆

Notes

Goals for Today_____ Ⓜ Ⓣ Ⓦ Ⓣ Ⓕ Ⓢ Ⓢ

Muscle Group Focus _____ Weight _____ Date/Time_____

Stretch ○ Warm-Up_____

Strength Training

Exercise	Set	1	2	3	4	5	6	7
	Reps							
	Weight							
	Reps							
	Weight							
	Reps							
	Weight							
	Reps							
	Weight							
	Reps							
	Weight							
	Reps							
	Weight							
	Reps							
	Weight							
	Reps							
	Weight							

Cardio

Exercise	Calories	Distance	Time

Water intake _____

Cooldown _____

Feeling ☆☆☆☆☆

Notes

Goals for Today_____ Ⓜ Ⓣ Ⓦ Ⓣ Ⓕ Ⓢ Ⓢ

Muscle Group Focus _____ Weight _____ Date/Time_____

Stretch ◯ Warm-Up_____

Strength Training

Exercise	Set	1	2	3	4	5	6	7
	Reps							
	Weight							
	Reps							
	Weight							
	Reps							
	Weight							
	Reps							
	Weight							
	Reps							
	Weight							
	Reps							
	Weight							
	Reps							
	Weight							
	Reps							
	Weight							

Cardio

Exercise	Calories	Distance	Time
_____			
_____			
_____			
_____			

Water intake _____

Cooldown _____

Feeling ☆☆☆☆☆

Notes

Goals for Today_____ Ⓜ Ⓣ Ⓦ Ⓣ Ⓕ Ⓢ Ⓢ

Muscle Group Focus _____ Weight _____ Date/Time_____

Stretch ◯ Warm-Up_____

Strength Training

Exercise	Set	1	2	3	4	5	6	7
	Reps							
	Weight							
	Reps							
	Weight							
	Reps							
	Weight							
	Reps							
	Weight							
	Reps							
	Weight							
	Reps							
	Weight							
	Reps							
	Weight							
	Reps							
	Weight							

Cardio

Exercise

	Calories	Distance	Time

Water intake _____

Cooldown _____

Feeling ☆☆☆☆☆

Notes

Goals for Today_____ (M) (T) (W) (T) (F) (S) (S)

Muscle Group Focus _____ Weight _____ Date/Time_____

Stretch ◯ Warm-Up_____

Strength Training

Exercise	Set	1	2	3	4	5	6	7
	Reps							
	Weight							
	Reps							
	Weight							
	Reps							
	Weight							
	Reps							
	Weight							
	Reps							
	Weight							
	Reps							
	Weight							
	Reps							
	Weight							
	Reps							
	Weight							

Cardio

Exercise	Calories	Distance	Time
_____			
_____			
_____			
_____			

Water intake _____

Cooldown _____

Feeling ☆☆☆☆☆

Notes

Goals for Today_____ Ⓜ Ⓣ Ⓦ Ⓣ Ⓕ Ⓢ Ⓢ

Muscle Group Focus _____ Weight _____ Date/Time_____

Stretch ◯ Warm-Up_____

Strength Training

Exercise	Set	1	2	3	4	5	6	7
	Reps							
	Weight							
	Reps							
	Weight							
	Reps							
	Weight							
	Reps							
	Weight							
	Reps							
	Weight							
	Reps							
	Weight							
	Reps							
	Weight							

Cardio

Exercise	Calories	Distance	Time

Water intake _____

Cooldown _____

Feeling ☆☆☆☆☆

Notes

Goals for Today_____ (M) (T) (W) (T) (F) (S) (S)

Muscle Group Focus _____ Weight _____ Date/Time_____

Stretch ◯ Warm-Up_____

Strength Training

Exercise	Set	1	2	3	4	5	6	7
	Reps							
	Weight							
	Reps							
	Weight							
	Reps							
	Weight							
	Reps							
	Weight							
	Reps							
	Weight							
	Reps							
	Weight							
	Reps							
	Weight							
	Reps							
	Weight							

Cardio

Exercise	Calories	Distance	Time

Water intake _____

Cooldown _____

Feeling ☆☆☆☆☆

Notes

Goals for Today_____ Ⓜ Ⓣ Ⓦ Ⓣ Ⓕ Ⓢ Ⓢ

Muscle Group Focus _____ Weight _____ Date/Time_____

Stretch ◯ Warm-Up_____

Strength Training

Exercise	Set	1	2	3	4	5	6	7
	Reps							
	Weight							
	Reps							
	Weight							
	Reps							
	Weight							
	Reps							
	Weight							
	Reps							
	Weight							
	Reps							
	Weight							
	Reps							
	Weight							
	Reps							
	Weight							

Cardio

Exercise	Calories	Distance	Time

Water intake _____

Cooldown _____

Feeling ☆☆☆☆☆

Notes

Goals for Today_____ Ⓜ Ⓣ Ⓦ Ⓣ Ⓕ Ⓢ Ⓢ

Muscle Group Focus _____ Weight _____ Date/Time_____

Stretch ◯ Warm-Up_____

Strength Training

Exercise	Set	1	2	3	4	5	6	7
	Reps							
	Weight							
	Reps							
	Weight							
	Reps							
	Weight							
	Reps							
	Weight							
	Reps							
	Weight							
	Reps							
	Weight							
	Reps							
	Weight							
	Reps							
	Weight							

Cardio

Exercise	Calories	Distance	Time
_____			
_____			
_____			
_____			

Water intake _____

Cooldown _____

Feeling ☆☆☆☆☆

Notes

Body Measurement

Date/Period						
Weight						
Body Fat %						
Neck						
Shoulders						
Chest						
Bicep Right						
Bicep Left						
Forearm Right						
Forearm Left						
Wrist						
Waist						
Hips						
Thigh Right						
Thigh Left						
Calf Right						
Calf Left						

Goals

Description	Deadline

Goals for Today_____ (M) (T) (W) (T) (F) (S) (S)

Muscle Group Focus _____ Weight _____ Date/Time_____

Stretch ◯ Warm-Up_____

Strength Training

Exercise	Set	1	2	3	4	5	6	7
	Reps							
	Weight							
	Reps							
	Weight							
	Reps							
	Weight							
	Reps							
	Weight							
	Reps							
	Weight							
	Reps							
	Weight							
	Reps							
	Weight							
	Reps							
	Weight							

Cardio

Exercise	Calories	Distance	Time

Water intake _____

Cooldown _____

Feeling ☆☆☆☆☆

Notes

Goals for Today_____ (M) (T) (W) (T) (F) (S) (S)

Muscle Group Focus _____ Weight _____ Date/Time_____

Stretch ◯ Warm-Up_____

Strength Training

Exercise	Set	1	2	3	4	5	6	7
	Reps							
	Weight							
	Reps							
	Weight							
	Reps							
	Weight							
	Reps							
	Weight							
	Reps							
	Weight							
	Reps							
	Weight							
	Reps							
	Weight							
	Reps							
	Weight							

Cardio

Exercise	Calories	Distance	Time
_____			
_____			
_____			
_____			

Water intake _____

Cooldown _____

Feeling ☆☆☆☆☆

Notes

Goals for Today_____   (M) (T) (W) (T) (F) (S) (S)

Muscle Group Focus _____   Weight _____   Date/Time_____

Stretch ◯   Warm-Up_____

Strength Training

Exercise	Set	1	2	3	4	5	6	7
	Reps							
	Weight							
	Reps							
	Weight							
	Reps							
	Weight							
	Reps							
	Weight							
	Reps							
	Weight							
	Reps							
	Weight							
	Reps							
	Weight							
	Reps							
	Weight							

Cardio

Exercise	Calories	Distance	Time

Water intake _____

Cooldown _____

Feeling ☆☆☆☆☆

Notes

Goals for Today_____ Ⓜ Ⓣ Ⓦ Ⓣ Ⓕ Ⓢ Ⓢ

Muscle Group Focus _____ Weight _____ Date/Time_____

Stretch ◯ Warm-Up_____

Strength Training

Exercise	Set	1	2	3	4	5	6	7
	Reps							
	Weight							
	Reps							
	Weight							
	Reps							
	Weight							
	Reps							
	Weight							
	Reps							
	Weight							
	Reps							
	Weight							
	Reps							
	Weight							
	Reps							
	Weight							

Cardio

Exercise	Calories	Distance	Time

Water intake _____

Cooldown _____

Feeling ☆☆☆☆☆

Notes

Goals for Today_____ Ⓜ Ⓣ Ⓦ Ⓣ Ⓕ Ⓢ Ⓢ

Muscle Group Focus _____ Weight _____ Date/Time_____

Stretch ◯ Warm-Up_____

Strength Training

Exercise	Set	1	2	3	4	5	6	7
	Reps							
	Weight							
	Reps							
	Weight							
	Reps							
	Weight							
	Reps							
	Weight							
	Reps							
	Weight							
	Reps							
	Weight							
	Reps							
	Weight							

Cardio

Exercise	Calories	Distance	Time

Water intake _____

Cooldown _____

Feeling ☆☆☆☆☆

Notes

Goals for Today_____ (M) (T) (W) (T) (F) (S) (S)

Muscle Group Focus _____ Weight _____ Date/Time_____

Stretch ◯   Warm-Up_____

Strength Training

Exercise	Set	1	2	3	4	5	6	7
	Reps							
	Weight							
	Reps							
	Weight							
	Reps							
	Weight							
	Reps							
	Weight							
	Reps							
	Weight							
	Reps							
	Weight							
	Reps							
	Weight							
	Reps							
	Weight							

Cardio

Exercise	Calories	Distance	Time
_____			
_____			
_____			
_____			

Water intake _____

Cooldown _____

Feeling ☆☆☆☆☆

Notes

Goals for Today_____ (M) (T) (W) (T) (F) (S) (S)

Muscle Group Focus _____ Weight _____ Date/Time_____

Stretch ◯ Warm-Up_____

Strength Training

Exercise	Set	1	2	3	4	5	6	7
	Reps							
	Weight							
	Reps							
	Weight							
	Reps							
	Weight							
	Reps							
	Weight							
	Reps							
	Weight							
	Reps							
	Weight							
	Reps							
	Weight							
	Reps							
	Weight							

Cardio

Exercise	Calories	Distance	Time

Water intake _____

Cooldown _____

Feeling ☆☆☆☆☆

Notes

Goals for Today_____ Ⓜ Ⓣ Ⓦ Ⓣ Ⓕ Ⓢ Ⓢ

Muscle Group Focus _____ Weight _____ Date/Time_____

Stretch ◯ Warm-Up_____

Strength Training

Exercise	Set	1	2	3	4	5	6	7
	Reps							
	Weight							
	Reps							
	Weight							
	Reps							
	Weight							
	Reps							
	Weight							
	Reps							
	Weight							
	Reps							
	Weight							
	Reps							
	Weight							
	Reps							
	Weight							

Cardio

Exercise	Calories	Distance	Time
_____			
_____			
_____			
_____			

Water intake _____

Cooldown _____

Feeling ☆☆☆☆☆

Notes

Goals for Today_____ Ⓜ Ⓣ Ⓦ Ⓣ Ⓕ Ⓢ Ⓢ

Muscle Group Focus _____ Weight _____ Date/Time_____

Stretch ◯ Warm-Up_____

Strength Training

Exercise	Set	1	2	3	4	5	6	7
	Reps							
	Weight							
	Reps							
	Weight							
	Reps							
	Weight							
	Reps							
	Weight							
	Reps							
	Weight							
	Reps							
	Weight							
	Reps							
	Weight							
	Reps							
	Weight							

Cardio

Exercise	Calories	Distance	Time
_____			
_____			
_____			
_____			

Water intake _____

Cooldown _____

Feeling ☆☆☆☆☆

Notes

Goals for Today_____ Ⓜ Ⓣ Ⓦ Ⓣ Ⓕ Ⓢ Ⓢ

Muscle Group Focus _____ Weight _____ Date/Time_____

Stretch ◯   Warm-Up_____

Strength Training

Exercise	Set	1	2	3	4	5	6	7
	Reps							
	Weight							
	Reps							
	Weight							
	Reps							
	Weight							
	Reps							
	Weight							
	Reps							
	Weight							
	Reps							
	Weight							
	Reps							
	Weight							
	Reps							
	Weight							

Cardio

Exercise	Calories	Distance	Time
_____			_____
_____			
_____			
_____			_____

Water intake _____

Cooldown _____

Feeling ☆☆☆☆☆

Notes

Body Measurement

Date/Period						
Weight						
Body Fat %						
Neck						
Shoulders						
Chest						
Bicep Right						
Bicep Left						
Forearm Right						
Forearm Left						
Wrist						
Waist						
Hips						
Thigh Right						
Thigh Left						
Calf Right						
Calf Left						

Goals

Description	Deadline

Goals for Today_____ Ⓜ Ⓣ Ⓦ Ⓣ Ⓕ Ⓢ Ⓢ

Muscle Group Focus _____ Weight _____ Date/Time_____

Stretch ◯ Warm-Up_____

Strength Training

Exercise	Set	1	2	3	4	5	6	7
	Reps							
	Weight							
	Reps							
	Weight							
	Reps							
	Weight							
	Reps							
	Weight							
	Reps							
	Weight							
	Reps							
	Weight							
	Reps							
	Weight							
	Reps							
	Weight							

Cardio

Exercise	Calories	Distance	Time

Water intake _____

Cooldown _____

Feeling ☆☆☆☆☆

Notes

Goals for Today_____ Ⓜ Ⓣ Ⓦ Ⓣ Ⓕ Ⓢ Ⓢ

Muscle Group Focus _____ Weight _____ Date/Time_____

Stretch ◯   Warm-Up_____

Strength Training

Exercise	Set	1	2	3	4	5	6	7
	Reps							
	Weight							
	Reps							
	Weight							
	Reps							
	Weight							
	Reps							
	Weight							
	Reps							
	Weight							
	Reps							
	Weight							
	Reps							
	Weight							
	Reps							
	Weight							

Cardio

Exercise	Calories	Distance	Time
_____			
_____			
_____			
_____			

Water intake _____

Cooldown _____

Feeling ☆☆☆☆☆

Notes

Goals for Today_____ (M) (T) (W) (T) (F) (S) (S)

Muscle Group Focus _____ Weight _____ Date/Time_____

Stretch ◯ Warm-Up_____

Strength Training

Exercise	Set	1	2	3	4	5	6	7
	Reps							
	Weight							
	Reps							
	Weight							
	Reps							
	Weight							
	Reps							
	Weight							
	Reps							
	Weight							
	Reps							
	Weight							
	Reps							
	Weight							
	Reps							
	Weight							

Cardio

Exercise	Calories	Distance	Time

Water intake _____

Cooldown _____

Feeling ☆☆☆☆☆

Notes

Goals for Today_____ Ⓜ Ⓣ Ⓦ Ⓣ Ⓕ Ⓢ Ⓢ

Muscle Group Focus _____ Weight _____ Date/Time_____

Stretch ◯ Warm-Up_____

Strength Training

Exercise	Set	1	2	3	4	5	6	7
	Reps							
	Weight							
	Reps							
	Weight							
	Reps							
	Weight							
	Reps							
	Weight							
	Reps							
	Weight							
	Reps							
	Weight							
	Reps							
	Weight							
	Reps							
	Weight							

Cardio

Exercise	Calories	Distance	Time	
				Water intake _____
				Cooldown _____
				Feeling ☆☆☆☆☆

Notes

[ ]

Goals for Today_____ (M) (T) (W) (T) (F) (S) (S)

Muscle Group Focus _____ Weight _____ Date/Time_____

Stretch ◯ Warm-Up_____

Strength Training

Exercise	Set	1	2	3	4	5	6	7
	Reps							
	Weight							
	Reps							
	Weight							
	Reps							
	Weight							
	Reps							
	Weight							
	Reps							
	Weight							
	Reps							
	Weight							
	Reps							
	Weight							
	Reps							
	Weight							

Cardio

Exercise	Calories	Distance	Time

Water intake _____

Cooldown _____

Feeling ☆☆☆☆☆

Notes

Goals for Today_____ Ⓜ Ⓣ Ⓦ Ⓣ Ⓕ Ⓢ Ⓢ

Muscle Group Focus _____ Weight _____ Date/Time_____

Stretch ◯ Warm-Up_____

Strength Training

Exercise	Set	1	2	3	4	5	6	7
	Reps							
	Weight							
	Reps							
	Weight							
	Reps							
	Weight							
	Reps							
	Weight							
	Reps							
	Weight							
	Reps							
	Weight							
	Reps							
	Weight							
	Reps							
	Weight							

Cardio

Exercise	Calories	Distance	Time
_____			
_____			
_____			
_____			

Water intake _____

Cooldown _____

Feeling ☆☆☆☆☆

Notes

Goals for Today_____ Ⓜ Ⓣ Ⓦ Ⓣ Ⓕ Ⓢ Ⓢ

Muscle Group Focus _____ Weight _____ Date/Time_____

Stretch ◯ Warm-Up_____

Strength Training

Exercise	Set	1	2	3	4	5	6	7
	Reps							
	Weight							
	Reps							
	Weight							
	Reps							
	Weight							
	Reps							
	Weight							
	Reps							
	Weight							
	Reps							
	Weight							
	Reps							
	Weight							

Cardio

Exercise

	Calories	Distance	Time

Water intake _____

Cooldown _____

Feeling ☆☆☆☆☆

Notes

Goals for Today_____ Ⓜ Ⓣ Ⓦ Ⓣ Ⓕ Ⓢ Ⓢ

Muscle Group Focus _____ Weight _____ Date/Time_____

Stretch ◯ Warm-Up_____

Strength Training

Exercise	Set	1	2	3	4	5	6	7
	Reps							
	Weight							
	Reps							
	Weight							
	Reps							
	Weight							
	Reps							
	Weight							
	Reps							
	Weight							
	Reps							
	Weight							
	Reps							
	Weight							
	Reps							
	Weight							

Cardio

Exercise	Calories	Distance	Time
_____			
_____			
_____			
_____			

Water intake _____

Cooldown _____

Feeling ☆☆☆☆☆

Notes

Body Measurement

Date/Period						
Weight						
Body Fat %						
Neck						
Shoulders						
Chest						
Bicep Right						
Bicep Left						
Forearm Right						
Forearm Left						
Wrist						
Waist						
Hips						
Thigh Right						
Thigh Left						
Calf Right						
Calf Left						

Goals

Description	Deadline

Thank you!

WE ARE GLAD THAT YOU PURCHASED OUR
BOOK!
PLEASE LET US KNOW HOW WE CAN IMPROVE IT!
YOUR FEEDBACK IS ESSENTIAL TO US.

Contact us at:

M log'Sin@gmail.com

JUST TITLE THE EMAIL 'CREATIVE' AND WE WILL

GIVE YOU SOME EXTRA SURPRISES!